Top 10 hacks for good sleep

Discover the secrets of restful nights

Kairos Somnik

Content

Introduction

Sleep is one of the most important activities of our body. It is the time when our body regenerates and our brain processes and stores what we have experienced during the day. A good night's sleep is therefore crucial for our health and well-being. However, in a hectic world where we are constantly under pressure and faced with a plethora of distractions, it is often difficult to get enough sleep and to sleep deeply.

This little book is designed to help you achieve better sleep. We have compiled the top ten hacks that can help you fall asleep faster, sleep deeper, and wake up refreshed and ready for the day. Each of these hacks has been proven and can help improve your sleep quality. We will refrain from unhealthy methods such as sleeping pills or crude tips like drinking alcohol before going to bed.

No endless reading of countless pages. In this book, we will present these ten hacks briefly, without rambling, and explain why they work. We will give you practical tips and techniques that you can easily integrate into your daily life. Whether you have difficulty falling asleep, wake up frequently at night, or simply wake up tired and restless - this book can help you optimize your sleep.

We hope that you will consider this book as a valuable resource that will help you get better sleep and feel better. Let's now begin to discover the top ten hacks for better sleep!

The Importance of Sleep

Sleep is crucial for our physical and mental health. While we sleep, our body goes through various stages that are important for different functions. A lack of sleep can have serious consequences for our physical and mental health.

How Sleep Affects Our Body and Mind

• Sleep affects hormone production and the regulation of metabolism.
• A lack of sleep can weaken the immune system and increase the risk of diseases such as diabetes, heart disease, and depression.
• Sleep plays an important role in tissue and cell regeneration as well as strengthening muscles and bones.
• Sleep deprivation can also lead to difficulties with concentration, irritability, and memory problems.

How Much Sleep We Really Need

• Recommended sleep duration varies depending on age and individual needs.
• Adults need an average of 7-9 hours of sleep per night.
• Children and teenagers need more sleep, ranging

from 9-11 hours depending on age.
• Even though there are individual differences, sufficient sleep is important for everyone.

It is important to monitor our sleep and become aware of how we sleep. In the next chapters, we will introduce the top ten hacks to achieve better sleep and thus improve our health and well-being.

Hack #1: Relaxation exercises

Relaxation exercises can help you reduce stress and prepare for sleep. These exercises can help calm your mind, relax your muscles, and prepare your body for a deep and restful sleep.

Breathing exercises

• Deep belly breathing can help relax the body and calm the mind.
• One simple breathing exercise is to take a deep breath and then exhale slowly and completely. Focus on your breath and try to calm your thoughts.

Progressive muscle relaxation

• Progressive muscle relaxation is a technique in which you tense and then relax different muscle groups one by one.
• Start with your toes and work your way up slowly until you have tensed and relaxed every muscle in your body.
• This exercise can help release tension in the body and promote relaxation.

Yoga

• Yoga is a form of physical activity that can help you relax your body and calm your mind.
• There are many different types of yoga, but some of the best for sleep are Hatha, Yin, and Restorative Yoga.
• These types of yoga focus on slow and gentle movements as well as stretches that can help release tension in the body and calm the mind.

Meditation

• Meditation can help calm the mind and reduce stress.
• One simple meditation exercise is to focus on your breath and calm your mind.
• Another option is to use guided meditations specifically designed for sleep, which can help you relax and calm your mind.

Relaxation exercises can help you reduce stress and prepare for sleep. Try different techniques to find out which ones work best for you. Regular relaxation exercises can improve your sleep quality and prepare you for restful sleep.

Hack #2: Creating the right sleep environment

A comfortable sleep environment can help you sleep better and feel more rested in the morning. Here are some tips for creating the perfect sleep environment:

Darkness

• Darkness is important to prepare the body for sleep and regulate the sleep cycle.
• Use blackout curtains or blinds to minimize external light influences.
• Avoid electronic devices that emit blue light, as this can disrupt melatonin production.

Temperature

• A comfortable room temperature can help you fall asleep faster and sleep more deeply.
• The ideal sleep temperature is between 16-20 degrees Celsius.
• Use a fan, air conditioner, or heating pad as needed to regulate temperature.

Noise

• Noise can be disruptive and affect sleep.

• Use earplugs or a sound machine to block or drown out unwanted noise.

• Alternatively, you can also use soothing sounds like white noise, ocean waves, or nature sounds to help you fall asleep.

Bed and bedding

• A comfortable bed and the right bedding can help you sleep better.

• Choose a mattress and pillows that meet your comfort needs.

• Use breathable and comfortable bedding to avoid overheating or discomfort.

Smell and scents

• Certain scents can have a calming and relaxing effect and help you fall asleep.

• Lavender, chamomile, and vanilla are scents that are often used in bedroom diffusers or candles.

• Avoid scents that are too strong or unpleasant and may disrupt your sleep.

A pleasant sleeping environment can help you sleep better and feel more refreshed in the morning. Try these tips to optimize your sleeping environment and achieve a deeper and more restful sleep.

Hack #3: Introducing Sleep Rituals

Sleep rituals can help relax the mind and body and make the transition from wakefulness to sleep easier. Here are some ideas for sleep rituals:

Relaxation exercises

• Relaxation exercises such as yoga, meditation, or progressive muscle relaxation can help calm the mind and body.
• Try out which exercises work best for you and incorporate them into your daily routine.

A warm bath or shower

• A warm bath or shower before bedtime can help relax the muscles and prepare the body for sleep.
• Feel free to use calming essential oils to enhance the bathing experience.

Reading or journaling

• Reading or journaling can help calm the mind and make the transition from wakefulness to sleep easier.
• However, avoid reading exciting material as it can keep the mind active.

Drinking a cup of calming tea

• Calming teas such as chamomile, valerian, or passionflower can help relax the mind and body and promote sleep.
• However, avoid caffeine-containing drinks such as coffee or tea before bedtime as they can disrupt sleep.

Avoiding electronics

• Electronic devices such as smartphones, tablets, and TVs can keep the mind active and disrupt the production of melatonin.
• Try to avoid these devices at least an hour before bedtime and instead choose calming activities.

Sleep rituals can help relax the mind and body and make the transition from wakefulness to sleep easier. Try out some of these tips and find out which ones work best for you. Incorporate them into your daily routine to improve your sleep quality.

Hack #4: The Right Nutrition

A balanced diet can help improve sleep quality. Here are some tips for the right nutrition to sleep better:

Avoid heavy meals before bedtime

• Heavy meals can cause the body to be busy digesting and unable to switch to sleep mode.
• Eat a light meal at least two to three hours before bedtime.

Avoid alcohol and nicotine

• Alcohol and nicotine can disrupt sleep and cause sleep disorders.
• Avoid alcohol and nicotine at least four to six hours before bedtime.

Eat foods that are rich in tryptophan

• Tryptophan is an amino acid that promotes the production of serotonin and melatonin, two important hormones for sleep.
• Eat foods such as dairy products, chicken, fish, nuts, and seeds that are rich in tryptophan.

Eat foods that are rich in magnesium

• Magnesium is a mineral that is important for muscle relaxation and sleep.
• Eat foods such as green leafy vegetables, nuts and seeds, whole grains, and legumes that are rich in magnesium.

Avoid caffeinated drinks

• Caffeine is a stimulant that keeps the mind and body active and can disrupt sleep.
• Avoid caffeinated drinks such as coffee, tea, energy drinks, and cola at least four to six hours before bedtime.

A balanced diet can help improve sleep quality. Try these tips and find out which ones work best for you. Good nutrition can help promote healthy sleep and help you feel rested and refreshed.

Hack #5: Technology and Sleep

Using technology before bedtime can disrupt sleep and lead to sleep disturbances. Here are some tips on how to use technology to improve your sleep:

Use Night Mode or Blue Light Filters

• Blue light emitted from electronic devices such as phones, tablets, and computers can disrupt melatonin production and affect sleep.
• Use Night Mode or blue light filters on your devices to reduce blue light.

Use Sleep Tracking Apps

• Sleep tracking apps can help you understand and improve your sleep habits.
• Use apps that record your sleep cycle and provide you with information on how long you sleep and how often you wake up.

Use White Noise Generators or Music

• White noise generators or soothing music can help calm the mind and promote sleep.
• Use apps or devices that can play white noise generators or soothing music.

Avoid Technology in the Bedroom

• Avoid using technology such as televisions, computers, and phones in the bedroom.
• Make sure your bedroom is a quiet, dark, and relaxing space dedicated solely to sleep.

Avoid Using Technology Shortly Before Bedtime

• Avoid using technology at least one hour before bedtime.
• Instead, use relaxation exercises, read a book, or listen to soothing music to relax the mind and body.

The use of technology can disrupt sleep, but by following these tips, you can use technology to improve your sleep. Try out these techniques and find out which ones work best for you.

Hack #6: Structuring your day properly

A well-structured daily routine can help prepare your body and mind for a restful night's sleep. Here are some tips on how to structure your day properly:

Establish a consistent wake-up time

• A regular wake-up time can help your body develop a natural sleep-wake cycle.
• Try to wake up at the same time every day, even on weekends.

Exercise regularly

• Regular exercise can help reduce stress and prepare the body for restful sleep.
• Incorporate regular activities into your daily routine, such as walks, yoga, or sports.

Avoid excessive caffeine consumption

• Caffeine can disrupt sleep and affect sleep quality.
• Limit your caffeine intake and avoid consuming caffeine in the afternoon and evening.

Schedule time for relaxation and stress reduction

• Stress can disrupt sleep and lead to sleep disorders.
• Schedule time for relaxation exercises like meditation

or breathing techniques, as well as for hobbies or activities that bring you joy.

Avoid heavy meals before bedtime

• Heavy meals can burden the body and disrupt sleep.
• Eat light meals in the evening and avoid large meals just before bedtime.

Create a relaxing sleep environment

• Create a sleep environment that is quiet, dark, and cool.
• Use soothing scents or essential oils and make sure your bed and bedding are comfortable.

A well-structured daily routine can help prepare your body and mind for restful sleep. Try these tips and adjust them to your individual needs to achieve the best possible sleep quality.

Hack #7: Reducing Stress

Stress is one of the most common reasons for sleep problems. When you are stressed, it can be difficult to switch off and find a peaceful sleep. Here are some tips on how to reduce stress and prepare your body for a restful night's sleep:

Identify your stressors

• Try to figure out what triggers stress for you. It could be specific situations, people, or tasks.
• When you identify your stressors, you can develop strategies to manage them.

Learn relaxation techniques

• Relaxation techniques like progressive muscle relaxation, autogenic training, or yoga can help reduce stress and prepare the body for sleep.
• Try different techniques and find out what works best for you.

Make time for yourself

• Regularly take time for yourself to relax and recharge.
• Read a book, listen to music, or take a walk. Do something that brings you joy and relaxes you.

Reduce your commitments

• Consider whether you can reduce your commitments to reduce stress.
• Delegate tasks, say "no" to commitments that you don't want to fulfill, and make room for things that are important to you.

Write down your thoughts

• When you feel stressed, it can help to write down your thoughts.
• Keep a journal or make lists to sort your thoughts and identify your stressors.

By reducing stress and integrating relaxation techniques into your daily routine, you can prepare your body and mind for a restful night's sleep. Try these tips and adjust them to your individual needs to achieve the best possible sleep quality.

Hack #8: Recognizing and Treating Sleep Disorders

Sometimes making simple changes to your sleep habits isn't enough to achieve good sleep. If you have persistent sleep problems, you may be suffering from a sleep disorder. Here are some of the most common sleep disorders and what you can do to treat them:

Sleep Apnea

• Sleep apnea is a common sleep disorder where breathing stops briefly during sleep.
• Possible symptoms include loud snoring, sudden awakenings, and daytime sleepiness.
• Treatment can range from lifestyle changes to using CPAP devices or other breathing support devices.

Insomnia

• Insomnia is a sleep disorder that causes difficulty falling or staying asleep.
• Possible causes include stress, anxiety, or depression.
• Treatment can range from lifestyle changes to medication to psychotherapy.

Restless Legs Syndrome

• Restless legs syndrome is a condition where you experience an unpleasant tingling or pain in your legs that can cause sleep problems.
• Possible causes include iron deficiency or certain medications.
• Treatment can range from iron supplements to medication to relaxation techniques or physical activity.

Narcolepsy

• Narcolepsy is a rare sleep disorder that can lead to excessive daytime sleepiness and sudden sleep attacks.
• Possible causes include genetic factors or autoimmune diseases.
• Treatment can range from medication to lifestyle changes.

If you suspect that you have a sleep disorder, you should consult a doctor to receive a diagnosis and find appropriate treatment. Successfully treating your sleep disorder can help you achieve better sleep quality and overall better health.

Hack #9: Natural sleep aids

There are a variety of natural sleep aids that can help improve your sleep quality. Here are some of the most commonly used ones:

Chamomile

• Chamomile is a plant that has long been known for ist calming properties.
 It can be consumed as tea or used as an essential oil in a diffuser to create a relaxing atmosphere.

Lavender

• Lavender is another plant known for is calming properties.
• It can be used as an essential oil in a diffuser or as a bath additive.

Valerian root

• Valerian root is a plant traditionally used to treat sleep disorders.
• It can be consumed as tea or taken in capsule form.

Melatonin

• Melatonin is a hormone naturally produced by your body to regulate the sleep-wake cycle.
• It can also be taken as a supplement to support sleep.

It's important to note that natural sleep aids may not be suitable for everyone and that you should always consult a doctor or pharmacist before taking them, especially if you are already taking medication or have health problems.

Hack #10: Maintaining healthy sleep habits long-term

It's one thing to have good sleep for one or two nights, but how can you ensure that you maintain good sleep habits long-term? Here are some tips:

Make sleep a priority

• Sleep should be just as important as a healthy diet and physical activity.
 Plan your days so that you have enough time for restful sleep.

Stick to your sleep schedule

• Try to go to bed and wake up at the same time every day to set your body on a regular sleep-wake cycle.

Maintain your sleep environment

• Keep your sleep environment clean, quiet, and comfortable.
• Regularly change your bedding and make sure your bed and pillows are comfortable and supportive.

Engage in regular exercise

• Regular exercise can help improve the quality of your sleep.
• Try to be physically active for at least 30 minutes a day, but avoid strenuous activities right before bedtime.

Don't put too much pressure on yourself

• If you have trouble falling asleep or staying asleep, try not to be too stressed or worried.
• Putting too much pressure on yourself can actually make it harder for you to sleep.

By following these tips and consciously striving to maintain good sleep habits, you can achieve better long-term sleep quality.

Conclusion

Good sleep is crucial for our physical and mental health. Unfortunately, many people struggle to achieve good sleep quality. In this book, we have presented ten hacks that can help you achieve better sleep.

From relaxation exercises and sleep environments to sleep rituals and natural sleep aids, there are many ways to improve your sleep quality. We have also discussed the impact of technology, stress, and nutrition on sleep and shown you how to positively influence these factors.

It is important to note that there is no universal solution for better sleep. Each person is unique and has different needs and preferences. It may require some experimentation to find out which hacks work best for you.

However, the most important key to success is consistency. By implementing these hacks as regular habits, you can achieve long-term improvement in your sleep quality.

We hope that the tips and tricks in this book will help you achieve better sleep and lead a healthier and happier life.